MEN
AND
SUPRAPUBIC
CATHETER
SURVIVAL
TIPS

I0171999

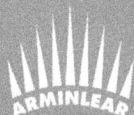

ARMINLEAR

Library of Congress Control Number: 2022940795

ISBN (paperback): 978-1-956450-18-7
(eBook): 978-1-956450-19-4

Armin Lear Press, Inc.
215 W Riverside Drive, #4362
Estes Park, CO 80517

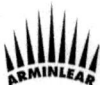

MEN AND SUPRAPUBIC CATHETER SURVIVAL TIPS

How to Be Superman with Your Catheter

Mathius Mack Gertz

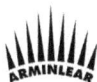

ARMINLEAR

KUDOS FOR SURVIVAL TIPS

"Suprapubic tubes (SPT) are often a necessary and temporary method of urinary diversion in the management of urethral stricture disease and surgically placed as part of the reconstructive process. A great read with helpful pictures to provide insight and helpful tips for men living with a suprapubic catheter for urinary diversion. Your book will be helpful and give many men insight into improving their experience while catheterized."

GLADYS Y. NG, MD, MPH
Health Sciences Clinical
Assistant Professor of Urology
Surgical Director UCLA Gender Health Program
Reconstructive Urology
David Geffen School of Medicine at UCLA

"*The prospect of experiencing catheter-ization as a result of a medical condition or procedure is at the very least daunt-ing. My fear and revulsion around the prospect of dealing with a catheter was almost phobic in its proportions; almost a Bucket List item to avoid it, but it was not to be. Thank God for my friend Mathius Gertz. His reassurance, and more, his booklet on the subject helped me deal with it with grace and dignity. He covers EVERY aspect of living with a catheter you can think of and many you wouldn't, because he's lived it and figured it out. This book is a must if you are facing catheterization whether it's a week or year. I couldn't recommend it more highly.*"

DR. JOHN MCGRAIL
Psychotherapist, author, *The Synthesis Effect*

"*Mathius Gertz' book covering the essentials of living with a suprapubic catheter is superb. Both informative and practice, Gertz delivers his message with the utmost empathy, kindness and understanding. It's a must read for any man dealing with this medical issue.*"

ROBERT C HAMILTON, M.D.

"I thought Men and Suprapubic Catheter Survival Tips *was excellent!!!*

As a general urologist with over 20 years of experience in private practice, I highly recommend Mr. Gertz's Men and Suprapubic Catheter Survival Tips. *Despite our expertise as surgeons, it is quite apparent that the urology community has fallen short on educating patients on the real-life issues associated with the long-term management of the SPT. This book does an excellent job of identifying these problems, and offers simple, practical, ingenious solutions that simply go overlooked in a busy urology practice. I think the recommendations are very medically sound, and I would highly recommend it for all my future patients who may need a long-term suprapubic tube. Very well done!!!"*

DR. SHAWN BLICK
Valley Urologic Associates
A Division of AZCCC Phoenix, AZ

CONTENTS

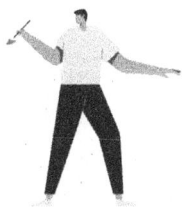

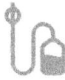

INTRODUCTION

By offering you tips on managing your current challenge, I don't pretend to be an authoritative source on catheters. I am not a doctor, nor am I a medical expert of any kind, although I have had doctors review this book to ensure my tips are helpful, never harmful. Consider me an average everyday middle-aged guy who can write and who had an accident—a fall. Through the !@#$$% architectural deck of a clients house. As a result, and in perfect health, I had to be fitted with a penile (or urethral) catheter and then a suprapubic catheter. During those ten months of having a catheter added to my wardrobe, I took a lot of notes, always intending to help other men who faced the same challenges I was having.

Everything I share with you here, I learned by trial and error. All the problems for which I offer you solutions in these pages I experienced myself while I was catheterized. I never want to go through this again, but since you or a loved one is currently going through this temporarily or permanently, I want to share what I learned to make your journey easier.

Nobody shared any of this with me—not the doctors, surgeons, nurses, or technicians. I am probably not the first man to try these solutions, but it seems I am the first to write them down for the benefit of others. Some of this stuff is embarrassing. Most of it is uncomfortable to discuss, and I suspect that most men don't.

In many cases, you don't discuss it because who could even imagine the solutions let alone the questions. My transparency and honesty about my experiences will hopefully make this episode in your life easier to bear. If you come up with some ideas of your own, let me know; I will add them to the next addition (see pages 83 & 84).

I believe that the dividing line in people is in their ability to exhibit kindness towards others. I made the effort to write this book out of kindness, and as a way to deal with the journey and give it a higher purpose. I am not trying to make money with my tips. After costs and expenses, royalties will be donated to charities.

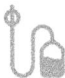

1
SLOW DOWN!

Living with a catheter—short or long-term—changes your relationship to time. It is going to take you longer to dress, undress, shower, and use the toilet. Don't get angry and frustrated. Make time to do what you need to do. Be proactive about appointments. Leave extra time to drive somewhere. Depending upon your age and health, it will take you between 30 minutes to one hour more in the morning to get ready for your day and another hour at night to get ready for bed.

Men are sometimes not as meticulous as women when it comes to hygiene. You may need to slow down and do all the things your mother taught you, and do them so carefully that she'd reward you with a cookie.

- » Wash your hands before handling the catheter.
- » Get a box of disposable nitrile gloves and put them on to apply ointments to the catheter site.

Your routines are vital. Get into them!

- » Shower at least once or twice a day.
- » Empty the trash in the bathroom regularly.
- » Change your bags every one or two weeks to a new one to minimize infection.
- » To save time in the morning, perhaps shave before bedtime instead.
- » Put out the things you need where you can find them.

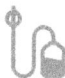

2
HOOKS IN THE BATHROOM

You are going to need a place to hang your urine leg bags and overnight urine bags that are safe and accessible. You probably don't want them out in plain sight if you can help it, so you might want to use folding hooks to "hide the evidence" when they're not in use

Take a look at your space and make a conscious decision about how you are going to hang them up and keep them clean.

Do you need help putting in a hook? Don't be embarrassed, call a handyman (or handyperson), and get it done.

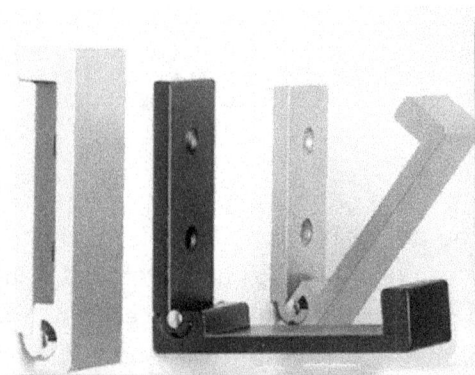

I found these at an IKEA. But I'm sure that a hardware store would have a version of it. Just look in the catheter section (kidding).

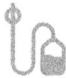

3
STATLOCK™

If you're just entering this rarefied club of catheter wearers, "statlock" is short for StatLock® Foley Stabilization Device and it comes with an adhesive anchor pad to affix it to your body.

No rule says you can't have more than one statlock on your leg and at roughly $5 each, they are not ridiculously expensive. You can use two on one side to direct the hose thru in an S-shape. You can put one on each hip so that you can shift which leg you attach the leg bag to on any given day or with the overnight bag, which side of the bed you want to sleep on. Get a few extra and experiment a little bit until you get them positioned in such a way that is most comfortable for you.

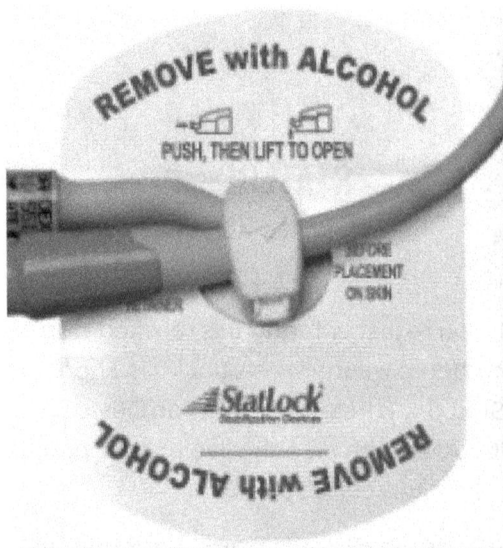

Since you have to have them on, think up some creative ways to use them in the bedroom once the lights go dim. They are the equivalent of having a carabiner attached to your body. You may be able to hook more to them than just your catheter tube. (See Chapter 23)

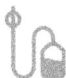

4
ANTIBIOTIC OINTMENT

Most surgeons and hospitals will tell you to put this on the opening where the tube comes out. I recommend that you get a triple antibiotic ointment with pain reliever. Most pharmacies have a store brand version.

The pain reliever does just what it says and can also help with the itching you will likely have. It does a good job of reducing the discomfort, especially when the catheter is new.

If you are allergic or sensitive to any of the ingredients in the triple antibiotic, I suggest using a lidocaine spray.

Lidocaine is a local anesthetic and the spray makes it easy to get it onto your latex or nitrile glove-covered hands. By applying it this way to the opening you won't get the little sting that can come with spraying directly on the opening. In all cases, check with your doctor first if you are unsure or concerned about using any of the over-the-counter antibiotic or numbing products.

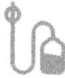

5
UNDERWEAR

One of the biggest problems for men with a suprapubic catheter is tenderness at the insertion site compounded by the risk of infection. The main culprit: men's underwear. We usually use underwear that has an elastic band and fits tight on the waist or hips. This will not work with a suprapubic catheter. It will be uncomfortable and will induce tenderness and infection.

I tried everything and finally came up with a solution. Women's underwear! The style of underwear known as "boyshorts" is usually perfect. Fruit of the Loom makes a good one. If you wear a medium in men's underwear, you will probably need a size large in women's. So, whatever size you wear, figure a size up or two and take it from there.

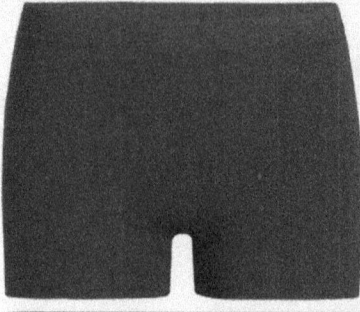

Consider going to the store with your wife or girlfriend. It gives them an opportunity to do something to help you and feel useful to you. If you don't have one, this may be a great way to deepen your friendship with a woman. She will be flattered that you trusted her with your secret.

Why does this work? Women are always sensitive to panty lines showing through their clothes. So, designers figured out how to make women's underwear that stays up without a tight bulky waistband. This is precisely what you need with a suprapubic catheter. If you don't get enough support for your genitals with the boy shorts, you can buy some women's hipster underwear and wear them instead of or over the boy shorts.

Women's hipster underwear is another type of seamless underwear that doesn't bind. Remember to size up for maximum comfort. Also, keep in mind that women's panties are thinner than male briefs. Wearing two pairs, such as a combination of boy shorts and hipsters, won't feel bulky to most men. Mix and match, front or back until you find a combination that works for you. The important point is no tight, wide, or elastic waistbands. Stay loose.

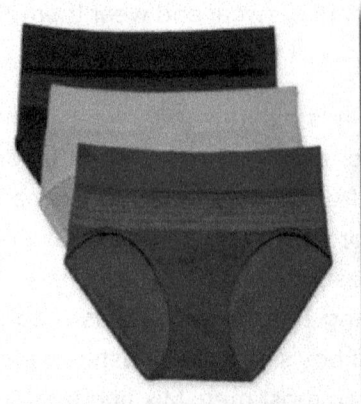

"Boy, boy, crazy boy. Stay loose boy." from the song Cool *in* West Side Story

It's going to look like the underwear won't stay up cause it has little or no elastic at the waist. Trust me; it will work. The fabric, even though it is 100 percent cotton, is designed to stretch and hug the body gently. Depending on your physique, they sometimes work better and are more comfortable if you turn them around and wear them backward.

Are you uptight about wearing ladies' underpants because you are worried about what people will think about you if you get into a car accident? Get over it. You have a catheter coming out of your abdomen. Who cares about the panties?

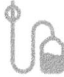

6
DRESSINGS

After the surgery, the hospital gives you a handful of sterile dressings to keep over the hole where the catheter comes out. For the first week, that's okay. After that, it becomes a pain in the neck. Trying to keep it on the wound while you are walking is difficult and uncomfortable. You have to attach it to your body with paper tape, and the hose moving around under it rubs. The dressing gets soiled from the wound's secretions, so you are constantly replacing it. The dressing is bulky and the process of replacing it is cumbersome. And there is no cheap way to do this: Sterile dressings in the supply you need are expensive at either the pharmacy or a surgical supply store.

An early solution I devised was to attach the dressings to the panties. But they weren't made to adhere to the fabric, so they didn't stick very well.

Then I got a better idea.

I tried using women's panty liners, and then I considered men's underwear liners for incontinence. Even though they are clean, they aren't sterile. The question is: Does that make a difference?

Let's look at the comfort factor first. Both worked well except that in both cases, the material they were made from wasn't designed to be soft enough to rub up against a raw wound.

From the perspective of safety, I found out that a well-regarded study had been done on "Sterile versus nonsterile clean dressings" to answer the question I posed above. The study included Coban tape, also known as Coban wrap, which is that soft elastic wrap that sticks to itself. Quoting the conclusion: "The panty liners, sanitary napkins and Coban tape studied were cheaper than, and had a comparable sterility with, the sterile gauze examined." (https://pubmed.ncbi.nlm.nih.gov/19554226/). Cheaper by about two-thirds, I might add.

So I kept experimenting with panty liners. I needed to find one made from a similar material as a cotton gauze or cotton surgical sponge. And I found it at the CVS pharmacy. Their store brand, CVS Health, has a pure 100 percent cotton panty liner that comes in four sizes. The smallest one, the "light," works perfectly. However, the trick to using the liners is not to attach them long ways from front to back but to attach them sideways at the level of your catheter hole site. They are soft, non-irritating, hypoallergenic, chlorine, colorant, and perfume free, breathable, and very absorbent. You won't even know they are there.

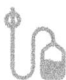

7
PANTS

Just like your underwear, your pants can't be too tight, or you are going to get irritated and be very uncomfortable. Many men just start wearing elastic waist, warm-up pants all the time. For one thing, many times, the elastic is still too tight. And another, who wants to wear warm-up pants all the time? So, you will either need to have your pants let out an inch, or buy some slacks or jeans that are an inch or two bigger than you usually wear.

Many companies make washable men's slacks that work great for this, and they aren't too expensive. Soft jeans that are too big in the waist also can work. You can search online to start.

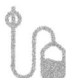

8
ADAPTIVE CLOTHING

Ah, ha! There is now another option; you may not find it at your local clothing store, but you can easily get it online. They are pants designed for people who have special needs and belong to a category of clothing called "adaptive." See, you've been telling people your whole life you had "special needs," now you can prove it.

With many people having medical or age-related needs that impact their clothing preferences, many companies have jumped into the business of making adaptive clothing, with comfort being one of the main design criteria. Adaptive pants often come with an adjustable waist, designed to expand and contract gently instead of grabbing you around the middle. Some also come with a Velcro closure to let you determine how loose or snug you want the pants at the moment, and a mock fly.

You can find adaptive dress pants, cargo pants, fleece pants, workout pants—just about any kind you need.

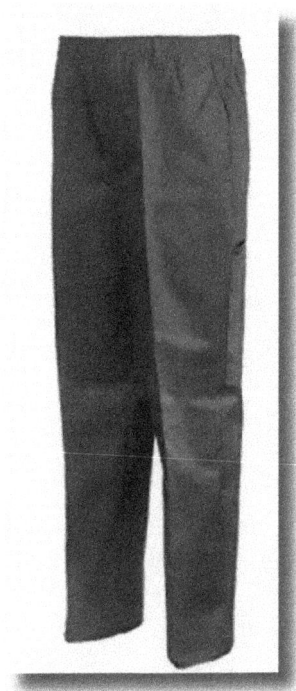

Most of these tips are for suprapubic catheters. If you are going to have a penile one for a while, you might want to get the pants a little bigger, or ask your doctor to let you switch to the suprapubic.

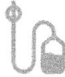

9
BELTS VS. SUSPENDERS

So now you have slacks that may be a little too big in the waist to create room for the catheter hose. The problem is you need a belt to hold them up. But if you use a belt, you create the same problems that you had before, or even actually make it worse. Here's my solution: suspenders!

Personally, I like the thin ones but not just because of the style. They are easier to get on and off, and when you have to drop your pants three or four times a day to empty your leg bag into a public toilet, I like to make it as easy, fast, and drama-free as possible. Thin suspenders are much easier to get in and out of than their wider cousins. Buy the ones that have four clips, not three.

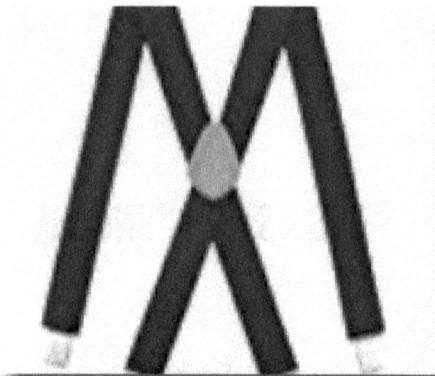

Three clips good. Four clips much much much better. You can also jazz up your wardrobe and get them in various colors.

So, what if you don't like the way suspenders look? Just throw on a sport coat, a jean-style jacket, or a sweater with a full zipper down the front and no one will know you have them on. You can find suspenders in tuxedo rental stores, some department or hardware stores, and online—lots of sites. Two black pairs is all you need, in case one breaks; unless you want to be more fashionable and get colors.

I grew to like suspenders so much that I now wear them all the time. I can't imagine why I would ever want to go back to wearing belts with a suit, especially when it is hot outside.

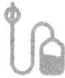

10
COFFEE, TEA, LIQUOR, WINE, AND BEER

You may or may not have been told by your doctor to avoid alcohol and caffeine. Regardless, let me share with you that these beverages affect your body so that urine output is more frequent. What that means is, if you want to reduce the number of times a day you have to empty your urine bag, cut coffee tea and alcohol out of your diet, or at least reduce your consumption.

You can skip this next part if you're not interested in the "why," but I know a lot of men who need convincing to give up that morning trip to Starbucks and the evening relaxation with a cocktail.

> » Caffeine is a diuretic, meaning it makes you pee more often. Coffee (or tea with caffeine) triggers signals to your pituitary gland to curtail production of the antidiuretic hormone (ADH). The result: Your kidneys don't reabsorb water, so you have to urinate more.
> » Any alcohol—beer, wine, or liquor—makes you need to pee more often because it scrambles brain signals to the bladder about when you have to urinate.

If you're a man of moderation and restraint, then go ahead and have that one cup of coffee and one beer. If one of either tips you toward wanting another one, though, just grab your water bottle. You need to stay hydrated—you just don't want to have an abnormally strong urge to go often.

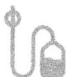

11
VITAMINS

You are going to find that exhaustion may wave over you. When the body is under stress, it takes a lot of energy to keep up a normal schedule. Therefore, you get tired, and your thinking can be a bit cloudy.

High quality vitamins can help a lot with your lethargy and lack of focus. Check with your doctor, who can do some blood work to determine what vitamins you need more of and what you already seem to be getting in good supply from your diet.

I found that a good quality multivitamin, Vitamin C, zinc, and B-complex should be your minimum vitamin regimen. Of course, you should check with your doctor first. Trader Joe stores, among others, have some good vitamins that won't break your bank.

You may also find it easier to drink your vitamins and electrolytes. Pharmaceutical grade products like Drip Drop, as well as comparable powders like Costco's Liquid I.V. and Pedialyte® all help keep you properly hydrated without causing "unnatural" urges to go.

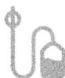

12
PLUGS

How do you switch from a night bag to a leg bag easily? How do you take a shower without wearing a leg bag or urine coming out of your catheter while you wash? How do you take a break from a leg bag when you go out to dinner? How do you have sex or sleep untethered to a bag once in a while? The answer is a catheter plug.

You can plug your catheter for long or short stretches. It is almost like having an extra hand while you are changing bags or for any other reason as well. Check with your doctor if you can use one for long periods or overnight while you sleep. But for convenience, ease, and a way not to have urine pour out of your catheter when you don't want it to, catheter plugs are a must.

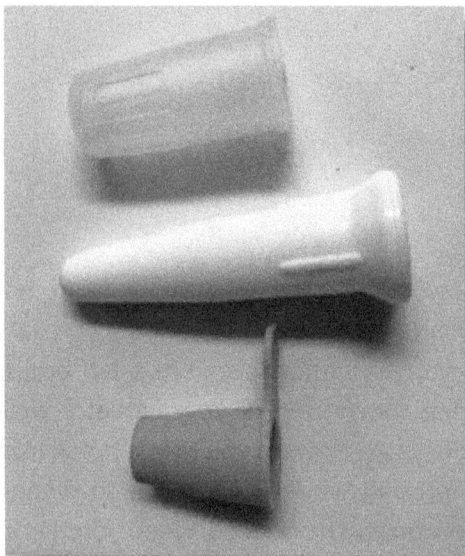

As long as you are catheterized you want to have these in your pants pocket everywhere you go. Everywhere!

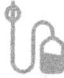

13
SOCKS AND LEG BAG IRRITATION

Sometimes the leg straps of the leg bags can be irritating to the inside of your leg or your scrotum. There are plenty of expensive ways to solve this at a surgical supply store. An inexpensive and effective solution is a 100 percent cotton ankle sock.

Among other vendors, The Gap sells packages of them. Just cut out a small hole in the toe, and you can slip the strap through it as you put on your leg bag. Then just position it where you need it. The pressure of the strap and your underwear will keep it in place. If it gets soiled, just throw it in the wash or get another one.

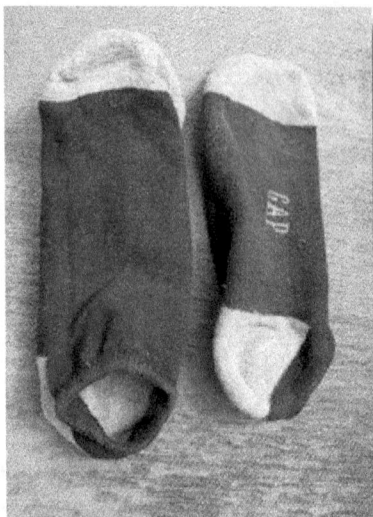

Duct tape is the miracle cure.If it still slips on you, use a small piece of duct tape to hold it in place. Back to the hardware store!

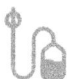

14
OVERNIGHT

When you wear a bag with a hose attached at night, it has to hang on something slightly lower than you, when you are sleeping or lying in bed. You could purchase a stand for this purpose. These are surgical supply items, and they are relatively expensive. Additionally, they look like medical equipment and are kind of hard to camouflage; one style hooks onto chair arms and bed rails so it quickly transforms your bedroom furniture into hospital furniture. If someone should come into your bedroom, say to get their coat at a house party, it would be obvious that someone in the house sleeps with a catheter.

Here is a simple solution and one that can be inexpensive, depending on your taste. Buy a valet stand. Ikea has a great one called MULIG , which starts as low as $12.99; it's what I used. However, there are plenty of others ranging in price from about $40 to more than $100.

A valet stand will not only do the job and not look like medical equipment in your home, but you can also use it to set out your clothes for the next morning. This will help save you time and aggravation during your morning routine.

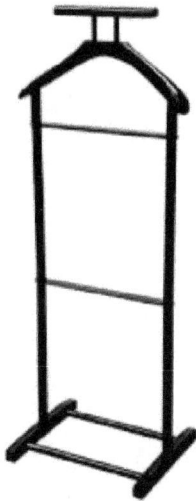

Having a valet stand is still a classy thing to have in your bedroom. You can also set your clothes out on it when you wake up and before you start the morning routine.

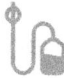

15
ALCOHOL PADS

Going back to item number one about hygiene, I want to focus on the use of alcohol pads. Use them liberally to clean the openings to urine bags that connect to your catheter as soon as you detach them from your catheter.

Nurses recommend you rub them for at least 15 seconds. Another option is to rub them and then fold the alcohol pad over and push it into the cap a little before you cap the opening to the bag. This way the alcohol pad stays in contact with the opening. You're going to change bags at least two times a day. Once in the morning, when you go from your night bag to your leg bag, and once at night when you go back from your leg bag to the night bag.

You should keep these openings disinfected as much as possible when they are hanging in the bathroom during the day or night. Alcohol pads under the caps that cover the openings can help a lot to reduce bacteria and infection.

Also keep a bottle of 70% alcohol in the bathroom with a spray bottle. Great way to make extra sure equipment and surfaces are clean.

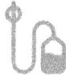

16
LEG BAGS

Hospital personnel may not tell you there are three sizes of leg bags. Hospitals generally only carry the large and small. For many people, the small one, which holds 500 ml (19 oz), is too small and the large one, which holds 1,000 ml (33 oz), isn't comfortable all the time.

Check with a surgical supply house to see if they have medium size bags with a flip-flow valve. They hold 750 ml (25 oz). You will have to change them a little more frequently than the large, but you may find the comfort is worth it. I highly recommend the ones with a flip-flow valve.

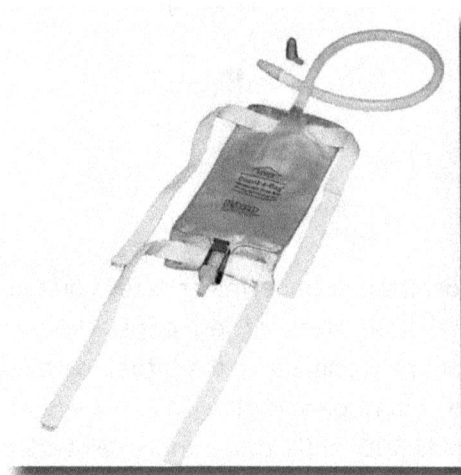

As Patrick Henry almost said,
"Give me flip flow or give me death."
Seriously, you want the flip flow.

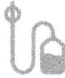

17
ACCIDENTS

From where I stand, there is nothing worse than having a leg bag detach from your catheter in public. It is embarrassing, messy, and stressful. The solution is to be attentive and proactive.

» Don't let your bag get totally full.
» Be aware of the nearest public restroom when you are out. Remember that almost every supermarket has a public restroom, and you don't have to purchase anything to use it.
» Make a point of going to the bathroom before you enter any

meetings that will last longer than 15 minutes. Pace your intake of liquids.

» Don't wear light-colored slacks. Stick to dark blue and black solids. That way, if you have an accident, your urine-soaked pants leg isn't as obvious.

» Keep an extra pair of pants or jeans neatly folded in a plastic bag in a small backpack in the car at all times. Keep a pair of underwear, socks, a few alcohol pads, and a package of baby wipes in there too.

» Make sure you use a backpack, not a piece of luggage, and take it with you wherever you go. A backpack gets less attention walking into a public restroom.

» Always keep a catheter plug and a leg bag cap (usually blue or green) in your pocket. Not in a sterile bag, just in your pocket. You want to get to them quickly, discreetly, and easily. With the plug, you can stop the urine from flowing out of your catheter, and with the cap, you can prevent the leg bag from overflowing. Even in public or in the car, if you have to pull down your pants partway for a moment and cap and plug, it will save you lots of aggravation and save the rest of your day. It is amazing how people ignore you and don't watch what is happening around them. Don't worry about what they are thinking. Just focus on yourself for the moment. Get the hole plugged! Did this happen to me? Yes! Right in the middle of a Nespresso coffee shop in Beverly Hills, CA.

If a detachment does occur, get to a restroom, and clean yourself up the best you can. I have noticed three things when it has happened to me. First, most people don't notice. Second, after you clean up, it dries out faster than you would think it would. Third, it doesn't smell terrible for a good few hours. So don't lose your cool. Just roll with it and don't let it happen again.

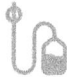

18
HIBICLENS® (CHLORHEXIDINE GLUCONATE)

Hibiclens® is an antiseptic, antimicrobial, and bactericidal skin cleanser without alcohol in it. It is 100 times better than hand sanitizer and it's available over the counter, commonly in the first-aid section of stores. Walgreens, Walmart, and Target are among the stores that generally stock it as well as pharmacies.

I recommend the 16 oz bottle with the pump.

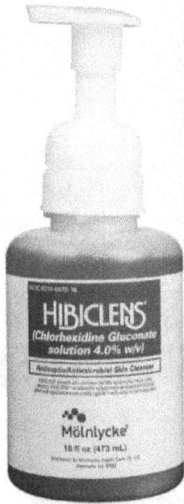

When you run out of patience and the routine wants to make you cry, Hibiclens will save you from becoming an infected guy.

Hibiclens is the best way that I have found to keep the area around the catheter clean and not irritate it or worry about soap residue. You can use it in the shower or out. Just follow the clear and simple directions. I kept a bottle in the shower to clean the catheter and the site at the end of the day.

Hibiclens is very effective against skin infections. You can even apply it to a washcloth or back brush to disinfect your body, especially if you have a lot of body hair, which tends to hold microscopic critters. It also helps with irritation from the bag on your leg.

I kept another bottle on the sink and washed my hands with it before changing bags or any other interaction with the apparatus. This helped to reduce infection and took up the slack when I just didn't have the inclination to put on another pair of gloves. The hospital will tell you not to touch anything without nitrile or latex gloves on. This works well when you are handling someone else's body, but not your own. It's just too much work and effort. You put on a pair, apply some ointment, take them off and throw them away, and then remember you forgot to do something. Hibiclens is a practical way to take up a lot of that slack and still minimize infection.

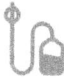

19
SHOWERHEADS

Having a showerhead fixed at or near the ceiling works for a lot of men, but women tend to prefer handheld showerheads to be able to direct water up or sideways to clean their vaginas.

Having a suprapubic catheter is not like having a vagina, but it does create the need to have the same flexibility to stay clean. It is essential that you can clean yourself in your pubic and anal areas, as well as at the catheter site and the catheter hose itself, better than you have before. You need to be able to rinse more effectively too.

Many showerhead products have two heads. One mounts traditionally. The other has a hose that attaches to the traditional head and is in a cradle that can be mounted on a shower wall at shoulder height. Choose one that is easy to take out of its cradle and return. Most also give you the option to change the water stream.

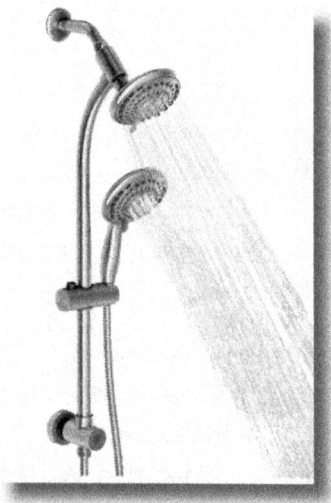

I recommend, if possible, not to buy the cheapest one you can find. You are going to be using this a lot. Get one that is well made and you really like and won't need to be replaced. Give him (or her) a name. Mine was Fred. We talked about catheters every morning. Made me smile.

You can find a great selection of shower-heads online and at home improvement hardware (again!), and plumbing supply stores. If you aren't up to installing it yourself, just hire someone to do it for you. It is well worth the money, and even if you no longer need to have a catheter, you will still enjoy having the new showerheads.

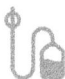

20
PENILE VS. SUPRAPUBIC

I had both types of catheters, a penile for the first two months, and then a suprapubic for the remaining months. Then I had both for a month after my surgery. It would seem that the penile would be better, easier, and less invasive. It doesn't require surgery, seems easier to deal with, and feels less permanent.

Many urologists will give you a choice while you are healing. Based on my experience, I recommend the suprapubic. It may seem counterintuitive, but the suprapubic is actually easier to deal with.

I had infection issues with both, so that wasn't a deciding factor. The suprapubic was just easier to work into a routine. It was also easier to work with because it was higher up and less irritating than having one in the penis. It also leaves your penis free to do some other things.

There is nothing about a penile catheter that is easy or routine. The suprapubic, on the other hand, becomes just a part of your daily grind. As long as you treat it with respect, give it the time it needs to be cared for, and don't overdo it physically, you will start even to forget it is there during much of the day.

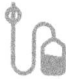

21
EXERCISE

I found a lot of articles about how there is no exercise you cannot do with a catheter. Then again, I found an article by someone with a catheter who described the agony of trying to run and cycle. In the more upbeat articles I read, supposedly even swimming is possible if you were to get a small bag and push it up under your swimsuit. You could probably also use a plug. Well, that wasn't my experience.

First of all, I was always on guard for infection, so I made a point of learning to keep the area when the tube enters your body dry. An infection can turn into sepsis very quickly. Trust me: This is really not fun. How do I know? That's right, from experience. (I can be such an arrogant idiot sometimes. So don't you be like me.)

In addition, I didn't want to damage anything nor accidentally pull the catheter out doing sit-ups. So, I tended to avoid exercises that targeted the abdominal muscles. This included swimming.

What I did do was develop a daily dumbbell routine using various weights. I started with two 5-lb weights and worked up to using a 20-lb dumbbell in each hand. I liked them over barbells because you can control them more easily and they take up little space. Buying a set that can adjust from 5 pounds to 30 pounds was perfect. I could store them and use them at home or on the porch if I wanted to. This took care of my upper body needs. My goal wasn't to bulk up. It was to maintain muscle, stretch, stay limber and not put on weight. A good routine could be done in 20 to 30 minutes.

For lower body I fast walked and climbed stairs instead of riding the elevator. A good brisk walk outside of at least four to eight blocks combined with a stair climb to your door gets your heart rate up and just enough blood flowing to burn some calories so that you will feel good about yourself—catheter and all. This would take all of 20 to 30 minutes, too. So, in an hour or less you can do a low impact routine that will keep you physically fit and contribute to a calm and positive state of mind. Believe me these two 20-minute routines will go a long way to keeping you out of depression, improving your self-image and keeping your digestion in good shape. And remember: Use my dressing tips, empty your bag before you start a routine, stay hydrated and know where the nearest bathroom is.

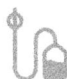

22
KIDS

I was concerned about being uncovered at home. I was afraid that my son would see me as being damaged or weak. The first time he caught sight of me uncovered with the suprapubic catheter and a plug his eyes got big, he grinned and said, "My Dad is a Borg!" referencing the half-machine race from the *Star Trek* series. That was all I needed. I wasn't embarrassed or insecure about the catheter after that. I was a Borg! I found that as long as I wasn't uncomfortable about the catheter, those around me weren't uncomfortable either.

(It doesn't make you less of a man,
Look, up in the sky.
Is it a bird? Is it a plane?
No, its "Supra-man".)

Depending on the age of the child, you can also introduce the topic of "having a difference" through one of the many kid's books such as James Catchpole's *What Happened to You?*

I liked being Borg-associated the best, though. Instead of just being different, I suddenly felt more interesting than "just" Dad, and even a little superhuman.

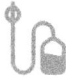

23
LOVERS

Like every other chapter in this book, what I write about here came from my experiences while catheterized. "To infinity and beyond!"

When it comes to intimacy, we are not talking necessarily about sex, although that is part of it. We are talking about being together in its myriad forms and configurations. Intercourse is part of that for sure. But intimacy is more than just sex, which for many people doesn't go on for hours, as it may in our imaginations.

For me, attraction begins with stillness and comfortability in one's own skin, an inner confidence, a creative openness, and verbal imagination. Having a catheter is very much like being Cyrano de Bergerac: a handsome and witty man in an imperfect skin. It's what you believe about yourself that matters more than what you look like. And what you believe about yourself, your self image, is also going to impact your physical recovery, your mental health and the quality of your life while wearing a catheter. For men, what we believe about the way we are seen by spouses, lovers or potential lovers matters. And I am about to be very direct. Please, read on.

Sexuality and wearing a catheter is very much a couple's game. What I mean is that it not only matters what you think about yourself, but it also matters what your partner thinks and feels about you. If she (or he, or they) scrunches up her nose every time you are half naked, it's going to be a hard emotional slog to be intimate, much less sexual, with each other.

Here are a few things to consider.

» Your catheter is, for now, a part of you. Don't treat it like something to be avoided.
» It's actually an exotic addition. Embrace the new you. If all of a sudden you were outfitted with a bigger dick, would you hide it and think of yourself as a freak? Probably not, so don't do it here either.

Many men who develop a belly in midlife find that their partners avoid touching their stomachs because it turns them off. They preferred you with a firm six-pack, or at least some firmness. It becomes a source of shame and decreases intimacy and sex—not because it is necessarily in the way of intercourse, but because it is an elephant in the living room, so to speak. An unspoken issue creating separation.

Catheters are much the same. If you avoid them, they become a source of division. But if you embrace them, they can be a source of positive amusement and eroticism. I see your eyebrows go up. Stay with me here.

In the world of sexual relations there are people labeled "vanilla." These are people who only have sex one way, usually with one partner on her (his, their) back or on all fours and vaginal penetration until his orgasm. If you are that rigid in your thinking, life with a catheter may be an impediment to intimacy. However, if you normally deviate from that even a little, you can actually broaden and improve your relationships with your new built in "sex toy." Have you ever used a vibrator? Okay, then you aren't vanilla!

I spoke earlier about plugs. This is a key component to intimacy and catheters because most of us don't have to wear the bag all the time. It's just a hose that can be tapped to the side with some paper tape, or if a penile catheter, folded over and secured to your cock with a condom. If you do have to have a bag on all the time, attach a new "fresh" unused small one with a flow valve before you meet for sex. If you think about it, most of us are averse to urine because of how we think it will smell. A new bag eliminates that fear.

A catheter tube and bag can be a source of verbal sexuality, erotic fantasy, suggestive manipulation. Many people like the feel of rubber, vinyl or plastic. Clothes and sex toys made out of them are very popular with many people. So, the feel of a rubber tube for many will be an erotic addition to your body. You can even accentuate it with rubber or latex gloves or other accessories. Perhaps make it the centerpiece of a verbal sexual fantasy during mutual masturbation. Or incorporate some silk or lace lingerie into the mix. Hmmm, rubber and silk. Yum.

Not everyone thinks of urine as disgusting. Some couples enjoy golden showers and have a more intimate relationship with bodily fluids. A catheter gives you the opportunity to play with those fetishes and fantasies in a new and different way. Most men and women who enjoy giving oral sex have experienced tasting a little urine and most are not turned off by it.

So having an abundance available is not necessarily a turn off.

Suprapubic or a penile catheter, you can still get an erection and have intercourse. How you view yourself matters more. Partners tend to follow each other's lead. So the fear of urine leakage is merely something to be dealt with proactively and with humor.

It's important to not see yourself as damaged or ugly. How about different or exotic? Reframe who you are in your eyes and your lover will be able to do the same. When they bring adult toys into a relationship, the first thing couples do is touch them and experiment. If you think of your catheter the same way, then you will help your partner not to avoid it but to embrace its being there.

As I wrote earlier, I believe for the long haul, that suprapubic is a better choice that a penile catheter. Let's assume you took my advice. You want to make sure you keep the hole where the catheter enters your body clean. So even during sex you should have some new clean gauze taped over it. One thing I liked to do was to take a clean pair of women's boy shorts underwear that I described earlier, and cut a slit in it so that my cock and balls can come through. I'd wear these during sex to help prevent roughness on the hole and also to prevent infection. Many lovers find men in women's underwear sexy. Others like the way "your package" looks coming through a slit in your underwear. Many people like to touch a partner "up underneath" some clothing, whether it's a shirt, skirt or underwear. Again, don't prejudge. Have a conversation. Move away from vanilla and enjoy a little mint chocolate chip! Think of your circumstances as an opportunity to try new things.

If you enjoy fantasy role play, incorporate the catheter into it. Make it whatever you want it to be. Become a *Star Wars* or *Star Trek* alien character. Perhaps you are outfitted with this special hose to overhear conversations or record fingerprints from a data base. Maybe, you are into Steampunk and you are half machine. Or from the future like The Terminator.

Perhaps now you are a sexual God? Or perhaps an escaped prisoner who has invaded a suburban home. The sky is the imaginative limit with your new built-in sex toy.

If you are already into fetishes with partners, having a catheter probably won't be a big deterrent. Open minded sexual partners tend to be, well, open minded. They appreciate change and erotic opportunities. You and your partner(s) just need to be a little mindful of this addition to your body when you get tied up, or spanked or blindfolded. With that said, some people will be turned off by your condition. That's what makes a horse race. Some people like only vanilla ice cream and others also like cinnamon chocolate or butter pecan. Take precautions against infection and continue to enjoy your kinky life. I promise if you do, others will too!

Finally, don't forget about romance. You can still go out to dinner, dance (perhaps slowly), take walks on the beach, cuddle on the couch, kiss and feel each other up.

If you're a long-time couple, use this as a catalyst to re-energize or expand your sex life. If you're single and dating, as long as you don't surprise someone with a catheter/bag situation in bed, you will find plenty of partners attracted to you. Female, male, or non-binary. Some will be attracted despite your condition. Some will see it as making you more erotic and appealing.

Communication is the key. Don't apologize. Just be matter of fact about it and talk openly. A centered, communicative, honest man is attractive to everyone.

How you see yourself is going to be a big factor in how others perceive you. Don't think of yourself as "less-than." You are merely in a new phase in your life. Whether it is temporary like mine was for ten months, or a permanent addition. You are still uniquely you. Your mind heart and body are attractive. There are, a handful, hundreds, thousands and more, partners down your street and all over the place that are hungry to have a partner like you, catheter and all. Even the greatest minds, entrepreneurs, sports figures, and beauty queens strike out sometimes. Rejection is not a tragedy or the end of the world. It is just inconvenient. Embrace your new uniqueness and more forward.

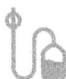

PARTING THOUGHTS

I hope you found this information practical, useful, and even amusing at times. I promise you that if you incorporate many of the survival tips I have shared with you here that your experience will be much easier to deal with. You will get through the catheter experience with less stress. You may, believe it or not, even find that it improves aspects of your life and your happiness.

I've always believed that men live three lives. The first one ends at age 30, the second at 60 and the third at 90. Anything after that are bonus years. In each life there are chapters. Your catheterization is a chapter you are in in one of those lives. You need to embrace and integrate it in. It doesn't have to be adversarial.

As I said at the beginning, I wrote this for no other reason than to save you from some of the challenges and discomfort (and ignorant mistakes) I went through. Please share this little book with anyone you know who might benefit from the information.

Finally, if you're inclined, write to me and share your experiences so that we can make it easier for the next guy. If your urologist, surgeon, medical center, or hospital wants copies, they may contact my publisher to receive a significant professional discount. (arminlear.com)

You are also welcome to contact me directly through email (SayWhyNotInc@gmail.com) or mail: PO Box 3707, Santa Monica, CA 90408.

Sending all good wishes to you!

And, may the force be with you and your catheter.

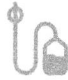

AUTHOR BIO

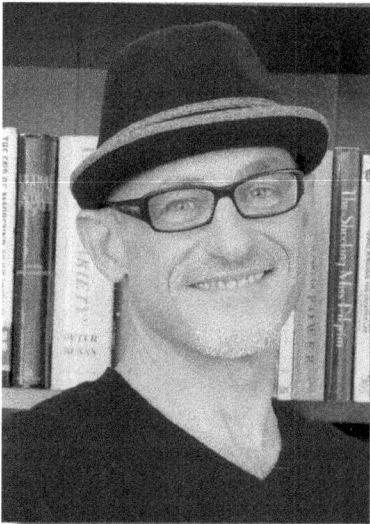

MATHIUS MACK GERTZ is a gifted storyteller and has been a life-long collector of experiences. Whether good, indifferent or bad, he has always preferred them to material gifts and enjoyed them all. . . one way or another. Wearing a catheter was not one of his favorites, but it was one experience that gave him a-lot of material and the motivation to share it with the world.

Born and raised in Brooklyn, New York, he lives with his family in Los Angeles, California. *Marc*, (his homage to a favored cousin) as he is known professionally in his mortgage business, holds an MBA, and an Accreditation as a Financial Counselor. He is a member of the Producers Guild of America and the National Reverse Mortgage Lenders Association, among others. You can learn more about him and his work at www.mathiusmackgertz.com.

"I hear you say 'Why?' Always 'Why?'
You see things; and you say 'Why?'
But I dream things that never were;
and I say 'Why not?'"
George Bernard Shaw
(1856-1950)

NOTES & INSIGHTS

_____

_____

_____

_____

_____

_____

_____

_____

_____

_____

_____

_____

www.ingramcontent.com/pod-product-compliance
Lightning Source LLC
Chambersburg PA
CBHW060341050426
42449CB00011B/2809